CHAIR YOGA
FOR
ELDERS
60

Cultivating Holistic Wellness through Gentle Movement and Mindful Exercise—Balancing Body, Mind, and Spirit for Vibrant Health, Flexibility, and Joyful Living"

Latasha R. Henry

COPYRIGHT

All rights reserved. No part of this publication may be reproduced, distributed, or transmitted in any form or by any means, including photocopying, recording, or other electronic or mechanical methods, without the prior written permission of the publisher, except in the case of brief quotations embodied in critical reviews and certain other noncommercial uses permitted by copyright law.

Copyright © (2024) ,(Latasha R. Henry)

<u>TABLE OF CONTENT</u>

Chapter 2: Getting Started

1. **Preparation**
   - Consultation with healthcare professionals.
   - Creating a safe and comfortable space.

2. **Choosing the Right Chair**
   - Features of an ideal chair.
   - Modifying existing chairs for yoga.

Chapter 3: Basic Chair Yoga Poses

1. **Seated Poses**
   - Gentle warm-up exercises.
   - Seated forward bends and twists.

2. **Standing Poses with Support**
   - Using the chair for stability.
   - Modified standing poses.

3. **Gentle Backbends and Balancing Poses**
   - Safe backbends for seniors.
   - Balancing poses with chair support.

Chapter 4: Breathing and Meditation

1. **Pranayama for Seniors**
   - Simple breathing exercises.
   - Benefits of mindful breathing.

2. **Guided Meditation**
   - Relaxation techniques.
   - Promoting mental well-being.

Chapter 5: Tailoring Chair Yoga to Individual Needs

1. **Adapting for Health Conditions**
   - Modifications for arthritis, osteoporosis, etc.
   - Working with limited mobility.

2. **Progression in Chair Yoga**
   - Gradual advancement in poses.
   - Setting realistic goals.

Chapter 6: Creating a Routine

1. **Sample Chair Yoga Routine**
   - Weekly schedule.
   - Integrating poses, breathing, and meditation.

Chapter 7: Enhancing Mind-Body Connection

1. **Mindfulness Practices**
   - Connecting breath and movement.
   - Cultivating present-moment awareness.

2. **Visualization Techniques**
   - Using the mind to enhance the yoga experience.

Chapter 8: Social and Community Aspects

1. **Group Chair Yoga**
   - Benefits of practicing in a group.
   - Building a sense of community.

2. **Incorporating Social Elements**
   - Socializing before or after sessions.
   - Organizing chair yoga events.

Chapter 9: Sustainable Wellness and Beyond

1. **Lifestyle Integration**
   - Incorporating chair yoga into daily life.
   - Encouraging overall wellness habits.

2. **Long-Term Benefits**
   - Aging gracefully with chair yoga.
   - Continuing the practice for a lifetime.

Conclusion
1. Recap of Key Points
2. Encouragement and Motivation

Review page

<u>INTRODUCTION</u>

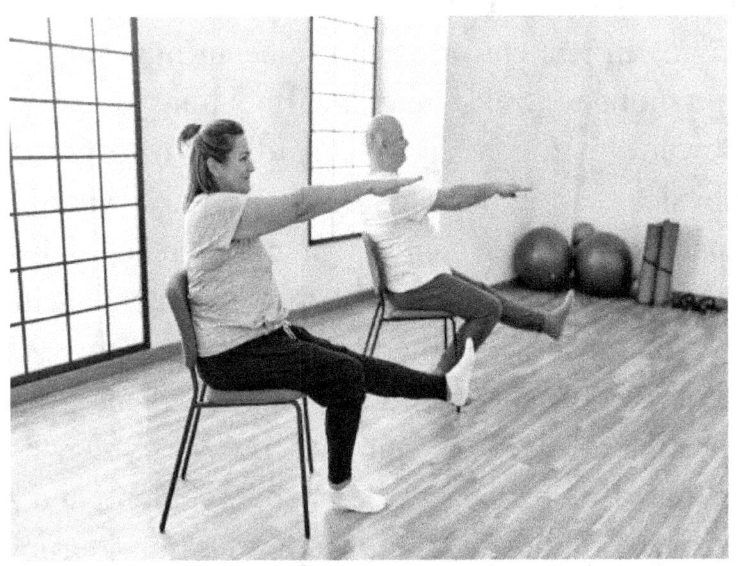

Welcome to **"Chair Yoga for Elders Over 60,"** a
comprehensive guide designed to bring the countless benefits of yoga to seniors in a safe and accessible manner. As we embark on this journey together, it's my sincere hope that this book serves as a source of inspiration and

empowerment for individuals seeking to enhance their well-being through the practice of chair yoga.

Purpose of the Book

Yoga, an ancient practice rooted in mindfulness and holistic well-being, has the transformative power to touch lives regardless of age or physical condition. This book is crafted with the specific needs of seniors in mind, recognizing the unique challenges and joys that come with the golden years. Whether you are new to yoga or have been practicing for years, "Chair Yoga for Elders Over 60" aims to provide you with practical guidance, gentle encouragement, and a wealth of knowledge to support your journey towards improved health, flexibility, and peace of mind.

Why Chair Yoga?

Chair yoga offers a gentle approach to the profound benefits of traditional yoga, making it accessible to a wide range of individuals, including those with limited mobility or health concerns. The use of a chair provides stability and support, ensuring a safe and comfortable practice. Through carefully curated poses, breathing exercises, and meditation techniques, chair yoga becomes a tool for promoting physical, mental, and emotional well-being.

In the pages that follow, you will find a wealth of information on understanding chair yoga, getting started with the practice, exploring basic chair yoga poses, and tailoring the practice to individual needs. Each chapter is crafted to guide you step by step, fostering a sense of confidence and empowerment as you embrace the transformative potential of chair yoga.

As we embark on this journey together, remember that yoga is not just a physical exercise but a holistic approach to living a healthier, more balanced life. Let's begin this adventure into chair yoga with an open heart and a willingness to explore the profound connection between mind, body, and spirit.

Chapter 1: Understanding Chair Yoga

What is Chair Yoga?

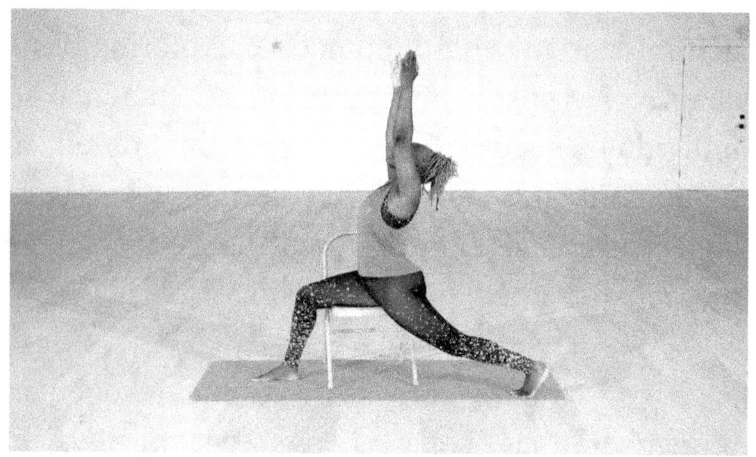

Chair yoga, a gentle and modified form of traditional yoga, brings the profound benefits of the practice to individuals who may face mobility challenges or prefer a seated practice.

By incorporating a chair as a supportive prop, chair yoga becomes an accessible avenue for seniors to engage in the physical, mental, and spiritual aspects of yoga.

Elements of Chair Yoga

1. Breath Awareness (Pranayama): Chair yoga places a strong emphasis on conscious breathing. By coordinating movement with breath, practitioners cultivate a heightened sense of awareness and promote relaxation.

2. Gentle Stretching: The practice involves gentle stretches that are tailored to meet the unique needs of seniors. These stretches aim to increase flexibility, alleviate stiffness, and improve joint mobility.

3. Strength Building: Although performed while seated, chair yoga engages various muscle groups, contributing to the maintenance and development of strength. This is particularly beneficial for supporting everyday activities and preventing muscle atrophy.

4. Mindfulness and Meditation: Chair yoga encourages mindfulness, inviting practitioners to be fully present in each moment. Meditation techniques incorporated into the practice foster mental clarity, reduce stress, and enhance overall well-being.

Benefits for Seniors

1. Improved Flexibility and Joint Health:
   - Chair yoga includes gentle movements that focus on improving flexibility in the spine, shoulders, hips, and other joints.
   - Enhanced joint mobility contributes to better posture and a decreased risk of stiffness and discomfort.

2. Enhanced Strength and Stability

- Chair yoga incorporates poses that target core muscles, the lower back, and the legs, promoting strength and stability.

- Improved strength contributes to better balance, reducing the risk of falls and enhancing overall mobility.

3. Balancing the Nervous System:

- The mindful breathing practices in chair yoga have a calming effect on the nervous system.

- Controlled breathing stimulates the parasympathetic nervous system, leading to reduced stress levels and a sense of relaxation.

4. Pain Management

- Chair yoga can be adapted to accommodate individuals with chronic pain conditions.

- Gentle movements and stretches may alleviate discomfort and improve pain management.

5. Cognitive Benefits:

- Engaging in mindful movement and meditation fosters cognitive function and mental clarity.

- Chair yoga encourages a positive mindset, reducing the impact of stress on cognitive health.

6. Social Connection:

- Group chair yoga sessions provide an opportunity for social interaction and community building.

- Shared experiences in a supportive environment contribute to a sense of belonging and emotional well-being.

7. Improved Circulation:

- Dynamic chair yoga poses can enhance blood circulation throughout the body.

- Improved circulation contributes to better cardiovascular health and overall vitality.

8. Enhanced Digestion:

- Gentle twists and stretches in chair yoga may stimulate the digestive system.

- Improved digestion can contribute to a sense of comfort and well-being.

9. Adaptability for Various Abilities:

- Chair yoga is highly adaptable, making it suitable for individuals with different abilities and levels of mobility.

- The practice can be tailored to accommodate those with physical limitations or health concerns.

The Holistic Approach of Chair Yoga

Chair yoga, with its multifaceted benefits, offers a holistic approach to health and well-being for seniors. The combination of physical movement, breath awareness, and mindfulness creates a harmonious practice that addresses the diverse needs of the body and mind.

As we continue our exploration of chair yoga in the subsequent chapters, you'll discover practical tips, step-by-step instructions, and a wealth of resources to support your personal journey toward improved health and vitality. Embrace the transformative power of chair yoga, and let it become a source of joy, relaxation, and rejuvenation in your life.

Chapter 2: Getting Started

1. Preparation: A Foundation for Success

Before you embark on your chair yoga journey, it's essential to establish a solid foundation that prioritizes safety, comfort, and a positive mindset. This chapter provides in-depth guidance on preparing both your physical space and mental attitude for a successful and enriching chair yoga practice.

a. Consultation with Healthcare Professionals:

-Individual Assessment: Schedule a thorough consultation with your healthcare provider before embarking on any new exercise routine. This step is crucial for obtaining insights into any specific health concerns or conditions that may require modifications to certain poses.

- Clearance for Exercise: Ensure that you have received formal clearance from your healthcare professional to engage in chair yoga, especially if you have pre-existing health conditions. This proactive approach ensures that your practice aligns with your health goals and medical considerations.

b. Creating a Safe and Comfortable Space:

- Clearing the Area: Begin by clearing the space where you plan to practice chair yoga. Remove any obstacles or potential hazards to create a safe environment. Make sure the chair is on a stable surface.

- Comfortable Attire: Select loose, comfortable clothing that allows for unrestricted movement. The right attire ensures that you can fully engage in the practice without any discomfort or restriction.

- **Appropriate Footwear:** If you're using a chair with wheels, ensure that it is stable and won't slide during practice. Consider placing non-slip pads under the chair legs to create a secure foundation.

c. Gathering Necessary Props:

- **Sturdy Chair:** Choose a chair without arms that allows you to sit with your feet flat on the floor and your knees at a 90-degree angle. Ensure that the chair is strong and supportive, as it will be your primary tool for the practice.

- **Additional Props:** Depending on your unique needs, you may want to have additional props such as cushions, blankets, or yoga blocks. These props can enhance comfort and support, especially during seated and reclined poses.

2. Choosing the Right Chair: Your Yoga Companion

Selecting the right chair is a pivotal step in ensuring a positive and effective chair yoga experience. Understanding the features of an ideal chair and learning how to modify existing chairs for yoga will contribute significantly to a supportive and safe practice.

a. Features of an Ideal Chair:

- **Stability:** The chair should provide a stable foundation, free from wobbling or instability. Stability is crucial for a secure and confident practice.

- **Comfort:** Opt for a chair with a comfortable seat and backrest. The goal is to support your body while allowing for ease of movement. A well-padded seat and supportive back contribute to overall comfort.

- **Height:** Pay attention to the chair's height. It should allow your feet to rest flat on the floor with your knees forming a right angle. This positioning ensures proper alignment and support.

b. Modifying Existing Chairs for Yoga:

- Adding Cushions or Pillows: If your chair lacks sufficient padding, use cushions or pillows strategically to enhance comfort. Placing cushions behind your lower back or under your seat can provide additional support during seated poses.

- Securing the Chair: If your chair has wheels, consider placing it against a wall or using a non-slip mat to prevent unwanted movement. Stability is paramount for a safe practice.

3. Mindset Preparation: Embracing the Journey

Embarking on a chair yoga practice involves more than just physical preparation. Cultivating the right mindset contributes to a positive and fulfilling experience. This section explores the mental aspects of starting your chair yoga journey.

a. Openness to Learning:

- Approach chair yoga with an open mind and a genuine willingness to learn. Each session presents a unique opportunity for self-discovery and growth.
- Embrace the learning process, acknowledging that every step forward, no matter how small, is a valuable achievement.

b. Patience and Self-Compassion:

- Understand that progress in chair yoga may be gradual. Patience is a key virtue in this practice, as is self-compassion. Embrace the idea that your body and abilities may vary from day to day.
- Celebrate small victories and acknowledge the efforts you invest in your practice.

Recognize that the journey is as important as the destination.

c. Setting Realistic Expectations:

- Establish realistic expectations for your chair yoga practice. Recognize that each day may feel different, and that's perfectly normal. Yoga is a practice, not a perfect, and progress is measured in personal growth and well-being.
- Listen to your body and honor its limitations. The goal is not perfection but progress and enhanced vitality.

In the subsequent chapters, we'll delve into the heart of chair yoga, exploring basic poses and techniques that will empower you on your journey to improved health and vitality. By laying this comprehensive groundwork, you'll be well-prepared to make the most of your chair yoga experience.

Chapter 3: Basic Chair Yoga Poses

Now that you've set the stage for your chair yoga practice, let's delve into the heart of the matter – the foundational poses that will form the core of your sessions. These basic chair yoga poses are designed to improve flexibility, strength, and overall well-being. Whether you're a newcomer to yoga or someone looking to adapt their practice to the chair, these poses offer a gentle introduction to the transformative power of yoga.

1. Seated Poses: The Root of Stability

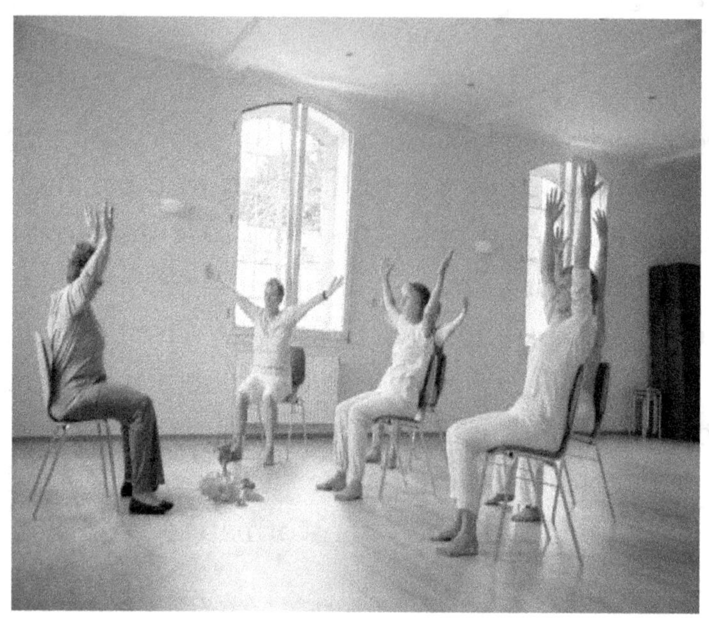

a. Gentle Warm-Up Exercises:

- Start your practice with gentle warm-up exercises to prepare the body for movement. Rotate your ankles, wrists, and neck to increase blood flow and flexibility. These simple movements will help ease tension and create a sense of readiness for the poses to come.

b.   Seated   Forward   Bend (Paschimottanasana):

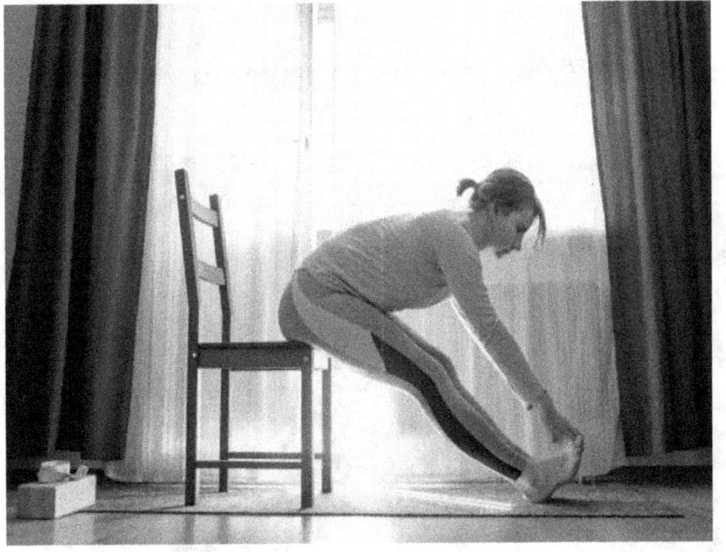

- Sit comfortably on the edge of the chair with your feet flat on the floor.

- Inhale, lengthen your spine, and as you exhale, hinge at your hips, leaning forward with a straight back.

- Reach your hands towards your feet, or if more comfortable, let your hands rest on your thighs.

- Feel a gentle stretch along your spine and the back of your legs. Hold the pose for several breaths, maintaining a relaxed neck and shoulders.

c. Seated Twist (Ardha Matsyendrasana):

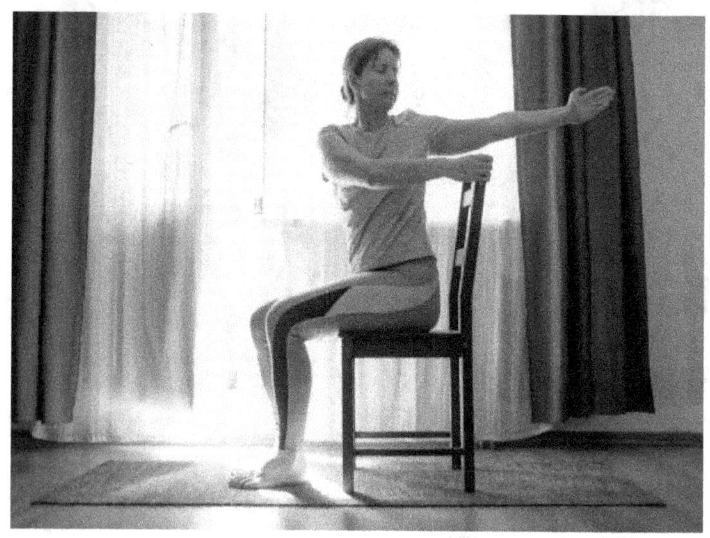

- Sit tall with your spine straight. Inhale deeply.

To - Exhale as you twist to one side, placing one hand on the opposite knee and the other hand on the back of the chair.

- Keep your spine long and your shoulders relaxed. Hold the twist for a few breaths, feeling the gentle stretch in your spine.

- Repeat on the other side.

d. Easy Pose (Sukhasana):

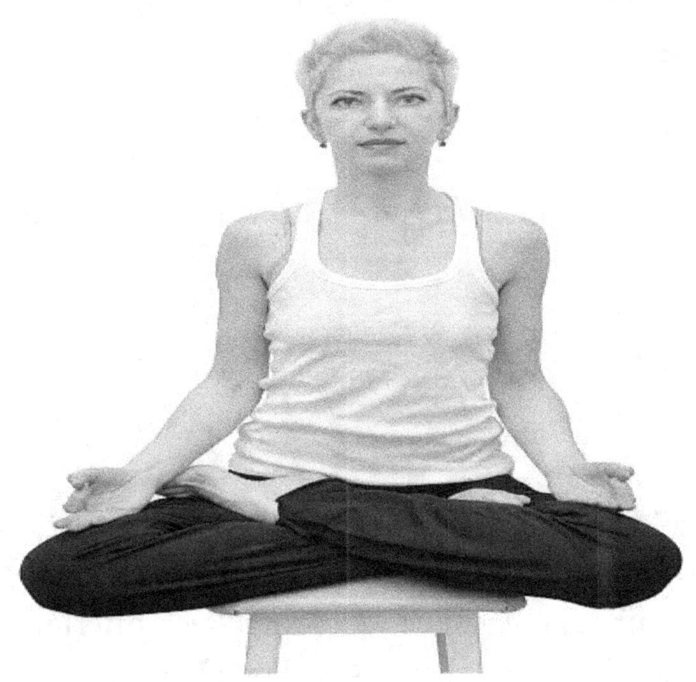

- Sit comfortably on the chair with your legs crossed, ensuring your knees are below your hips.

- Rest your hands on your knees, close your eyes, and focus on your breath.

- This seated meditation pose promotes calmness and relaxation, providing a moment of centering before progressing to more dynamic poses.

2. Standing Poses with Support: Stability in Motion

While seated poses provide a solid foundation, incorporating standing poses with the support of a chair can enhance your practice, offering a balance between stability and movement.

a. Tree Pose (Vrikshasana) with Chair Support:

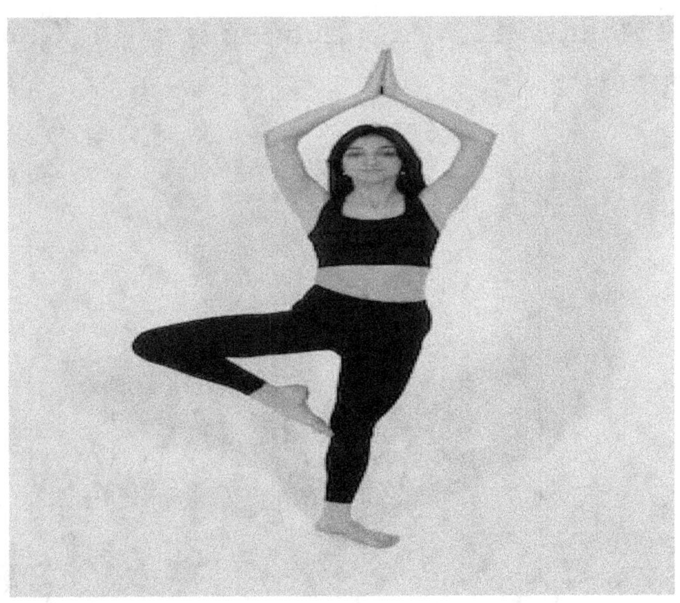

- Stand behind the chair, using it for support.

- Shift your weight to one leg, lifting the opposite foot and placing it against the inner calf or thigh of the standing leg.

- Bring your palms together in front of your chest or extend your arms overhead.

- Use the chair for balance if needed, focusing on grounding through your standing foot.

b. Mountain Pose (Tadasana) with Chair Support:

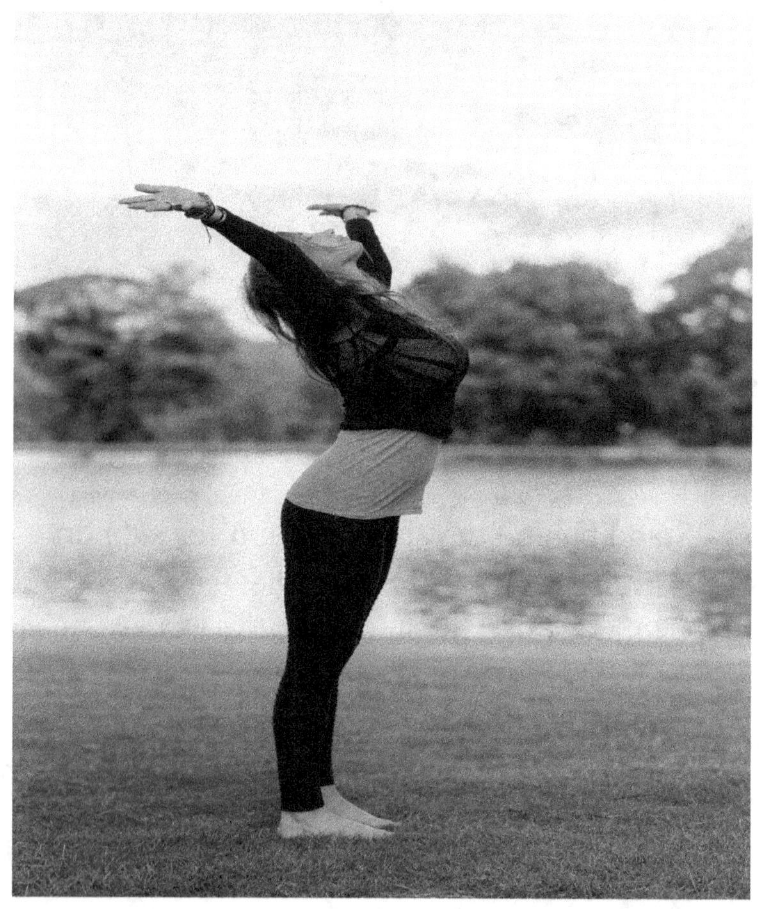

- Stand tall with your feet hip-width apart, arms by your sides.
- Engage your thighs and lift your chest.
- Use the chair for support if balance is challenging, grounding through your feet and reaching your arms upward.

3. Gentle Backbends and Balancing Poses: Cultivating Strength

These poses focus on gentle backbends and balancing movements, promoting strength and flexibility while ensuring stability with the support of a chair.

a. Cat-Cow Stretch:

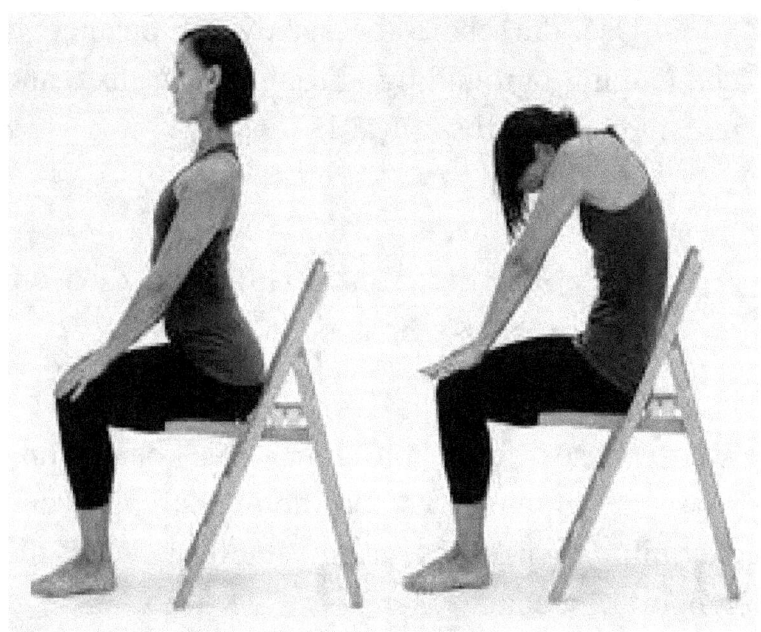

- Sit on the edge of the chair with your hands on your knees.

- Inhale as you arch your back, lifting your chest and looking upward (Cow).

- Exhale as you round your spine, tucking your chin to your chest (Cat).

- Repeat this flowing movement several times, coordinating with your breath.

b. Cobra Pose (Bhujangasana):

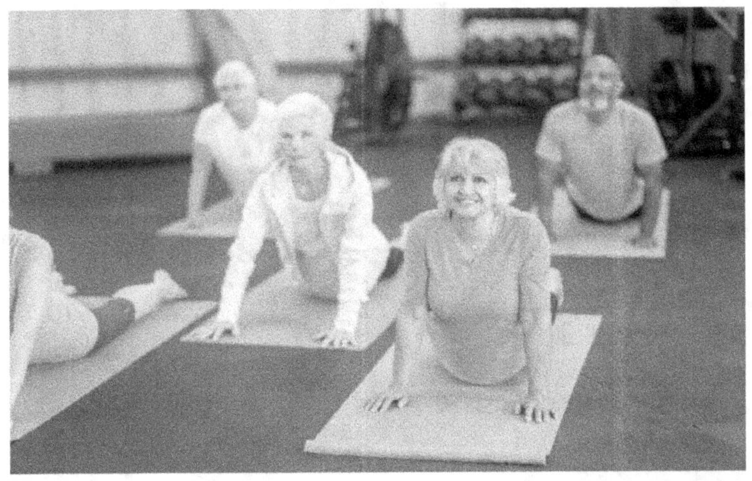

- Sit near the edge of the chair with your hands on your thighs.

- Inhale, lengthen your spine, and gently arch backward, lifting your chest and looking upward.

- Keep the movement controlled, and exhale as you return to a neutral position.

c. Bridge Pose (Setu Bandhasana):

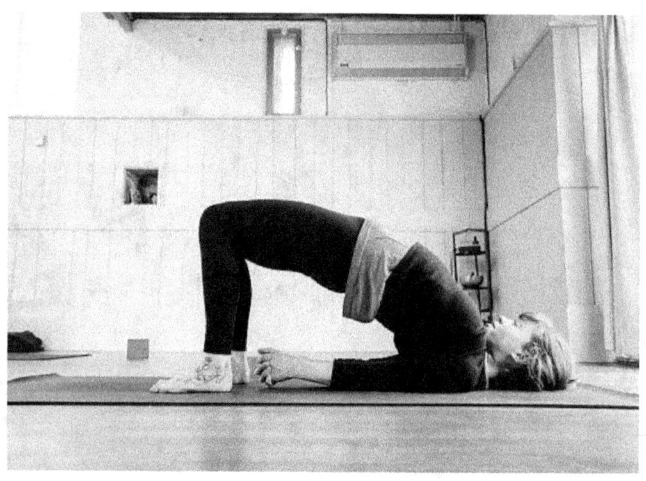

- Sit comfortably on the chair with your feet hip-width apart.
- Place your hands on the sides of the chair, fingers pointing forward.
- Inhale as you press through your feet, lift your hips, and open your chest.
- Hold the position for a few breaths, engaging your glutes and thighs.

4. Breathing Exercises (Pranayama): Nurturing the Breath

Breath awareness is a fundamental aspect of yoga. These simple pranayama exercises can be practiced while seated, promoting relaxation and mindfulness.

a. Deep Belly Breathing:

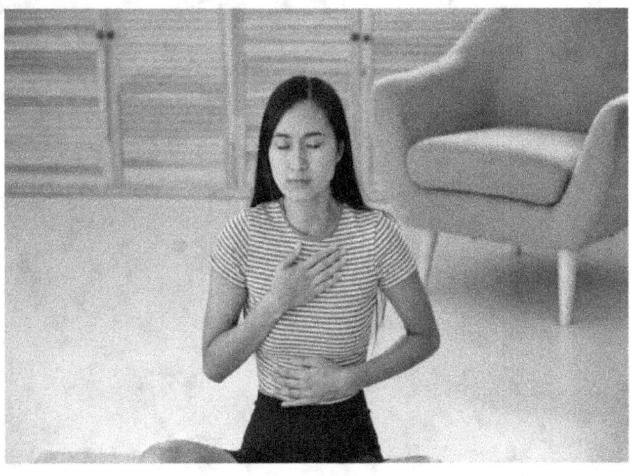

- Sit comfortably with your hands on your belly.

- Inhale deeply through your nose, allowing your belly to expand.
- Exhale slowly through your mouth, drawing your navel toward your spine.
- Focus on the rhythm of your breath, fostering a sense of calm.

b. Alternate Nostril Breathing:

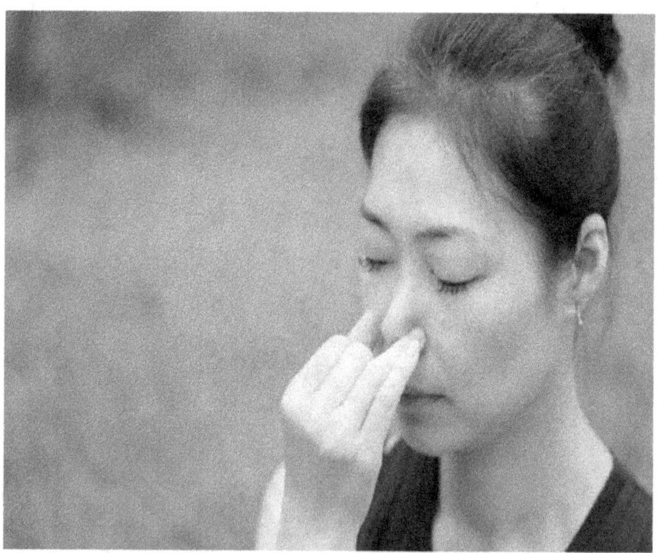

- Sit with a straight spine, using the chair for support if needed.

- Use your thumb to close off one nostril and inhale through the other.

- Close the other nostril with your ring finger, exhale through the first nostril.

- Repeat, alternating nostrils with each breath. This technique balances energy and calms the mind.

5. Guided Meditation: Journey Within

The practice of guided meditation in a seated position promotes relaxation, mental clarity, and a deeper connection with oneself.

a. Mindfulness Meditation:

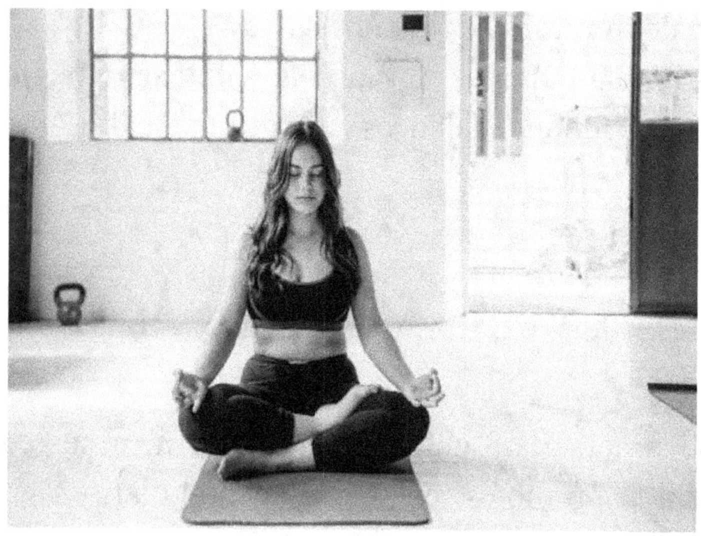

- Sit comfortably with your hands resting on your lap.

- Close your eyes and focus on your breath. Inhale and exhale naturally.

Allow your thoughts to come and go without judgment. If your mind wanders, gently bring your focus back to your breath.

- Feel the sensation of each breath, cultivating a sense of presence and mindfulness.

- As you become more comfortable with the practice, you can extend the duration of your meditation.

b. Loving-Kindness Meditation:

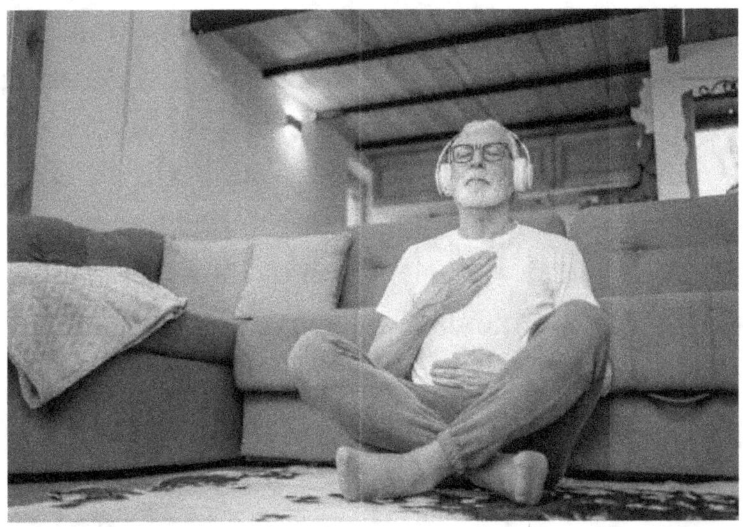

- Begin by sending positive and compassionate thoughts to yourself. Silently repeat phrases like, "May I be happy, may I be healthy, may I be safe, may I live with ease."

- Gradually extend these wishes to others, envisioning friends, family, and eventually all beings.
- This meditation fosters a sense of connection, empathy, and kindness.

In the next chapter, we'll delve into the art of tailoring chair yoga to individual needs, ensuring that the practice is adaptable for various health conditions and levels of mobility. This personalized approach will empower you to create a yoga experience that aligns with your unique requirements and aspirations.

Chapter 4: Tailoring Chair Yoga to Individual Needs

In this chapter, we delve into the nuanced art of tailoring chair yoga to meet individual needs. The beauty of chair yoga lies in its adaptability, making it an ideal practice for a diverse range of individuals with varying health conditions, mobility levels, and preferences. By understanding how to modify poses and sequences, chair yoga can become a highly personalized and inclusive practice.

1. Adapting for Health Conditions

a. Arthritis:

- **Modified Hand Exercises:** Start with gentle hand exercises, flexing and extending fingers to enhance joint mobility without causing strain.

Incorporate circular movements to promote circulation and flexibility.

- **Seated Leg Lifts:** Gradually introduce seated leg lifts, allowing individuals to lift and lower their legs one at a time. This promotes circulation without putting excessive stress on arthritic joints.

- **Gentle Twists:** Include seated twists with controlled movements to offer a gentle stretch to the spine, aiding in flexibility without exacerbating arthritis symptoms.

b. Osteoporosis:

- **Seated Side Bends:** Focus on seated side bends that engage the core muscles and promote spinal flexibility without requiring forward flexion, which may be contraindicated for individuals with osteoporosis.

- **Gentle Back Extensions:** Introduce seated back extensions, encouraging individuals to open their chest and maintain a neutral spine to strengthen the back muscles safely.

- Leg Strengthening Poses: Incorporate seated leg lifts and extensions to promote lower body strength, emphasizing the importance of building strength gradually.

c. Chronic Pain:

- Mindful Movement: Emphasize slow and controlled movements, ensuring practitioners maintain awareness of sensations. Mindful movement helps alleviate tension associated with chronic pain.

- Breathing Techniques: Integrate specific breathwork tailored to chronic pain management. Slow, intentional breathing can induce a relaxation response, reducing overall pain levels.

- Supported Poses: Utilize props such as cushions or blankets to provide additional support during poses, promoting comfort and relaxation.

d. Limited Mobility:

- Seated Poses with Support: Concentrate on poses where the chair provides stability, allowing individuals with limited mobility to engage comfortably in seated stretches that enhance flexibility.

- Arm and Hand Movements: Incorporate gentle arm and hand exercises that improve circulation and flexibility without requiring extensive movement.

- Breathing Exercises: Place emphasis on pranayama techniques, fostering a mind-body connection while seated, enhancing overall well-being.

2. Progression in Chair Yoga

a. Gradual Advancement in Poses:

- Encourage practitioners to gradually advance in poses, introducing new ones slowly and systematically.
- Provide variations to cater to different levels of experience and comfort, ensuring that individuals can progress at their own pace.
- Emphasize the importance of listening to the body and recognizing individual limits to avoid overexertion.

b. Setting Realistic Goals:

- Guide practitioners in setting realistic and achievable goals based on their unique circumstances.

- Celebrate small milestones, fostering a sense of accomplishment and motivating individuals to continue their chair yoga journey.

- Reinforce that progress in chair yoga is personal, and each practitioner's journey is unique.

3. Customizing for Various Abilities

a. Seated Variations for Different Poses:

- Offer seated variations for standing poses, allowing individuals with varying abilities to experience the benefits of each pose without putting strain on their bodies.

- Provide detailed instructions on how to adapt standing poses with chair support, ensuring safety and accessibility.

b. **Use of Props:

- Explore the versatile use of props, such as yoga straps, blocks, or blankets, to enhance support and accessibility during chair yoga.

- Provide demonstrations and instructions on how props can be utilized effectively, catering to specific needs and preferences.

c. Mindfulness and Adaptability:

- Stress the importance of mindfulness during practice, encouraging individuals to be fully present and tune into their bodies.

- Foster a sense of adaptability, empowering practitioners to modify poses as needed without judgment. Encourage a mindset of exploration and self-discovery.

Tailoring chair yoga to individual needs is a journey of exploration and adaptation. By understanding the considerations for specific health conditions, promoting gradual progression, and customizing poses for various abilities, practitioners can truly experience the transformative benefits of chair yoga in a way that resonates with their unique circumstances. As we move forward, the next chapter will guide you in creating a structured chair yoga routine, allowing individuals to integrate these personalized practices into their daily lives seamlessly.

Chapter 5: Creating Your Structured Chair Yoga Routine

Welcome to the chapter dedicated to crafting your personalized chair yoga routine. This transformative journey involves defining your goals, selecting appropriate poses, adapting them to your needs, establishing a consistent schedule, and tracking your progress. By following this step-by-step guide, you'll not only build a routine but also cultivate a deeper connection with your body and mind through the practice of chair yoga.

1. Defining Your Goals

a. Physical Health Goals:

- Take a deeper dive into specific physical goals. Are you focusing on increasing flexibility in your hips or improving strength in your core?

- Consider any existing health conditions and tailor your goals to address those areas that require attention.

b. Mental and Emotional Goals:

- Reflect on your mental and emotional well-being. Perhaps you aim to reduce stress, enhance focus, or cultivate emotional balance.
- Consider how chair yoga can serve as a tool for mindfulness, providing a space for emotional self-regulation.

c. Time Commitment:

- Determine the frequency and duration of your chair yoga sessions based on your schedule.
- Recognize that even short, consistent sessions can yield substantial benefits over time.

d. Holistic Wellness:

- Explore how chair yoga can contribute to your overall well-being, not just physically but emotionally and mentally as well.

- Think of your routine as a holistic approach to wellness, addressing various facets of your health.

2. Selecting Poses for Your Routine

a. Incorporating Warm-Up Poses:

- Delve into specific warm-up poses that cater to your body's unique needs. Consider movements that release tension in areas where you typically hold stress.

- Incorporate dynamic stretches that gradually increase blood flow and flexibility.

b. Main Pose Sequence:

- Choose a sequence of poses that align with your identified goals. If strength is a focus, include poses that engage major muscle groups.

- Ensure variety to keep your routine engaging and to target different aspects of fitness and flexibility.

c. Mindfulness and Breathing Practices:

- Explore various mindfulness exercises, such as body scans or mindful breathing, and select those that resonate with you.

- Experiment with different pranayama techniques, understanding how each breath practice affects your mental and emotional state.

d. Cooling Down and Restorative Poses:

- Personalize your cool-down section with poses that provide a sense of relaxation and restoration.

- Consider poses that facilitate gentle stretching and deep breathing to transition your body into a state of calm.

3. Adapting Poses for Your Needs

a. Personalizing for Health Conditions:

- Tailor your routine to accommodate any specific health conditions or physical limitations you may have.
- Work closely with the adaptations and modifications outlined in earlier chapters, ensuring a safe and effective practice.

b. Setting Intensity Levels:

- Develop different versions of your routine to accommodate varying energy levels.
- Create options for gentle sessions on days when you need a more nurturing practice and more dynamic sequences when you crave increased intensity.

c. Exploration and Experimentation:

- Allow room for exploration within your routine. Be open to trying new poses and modifications as your practice evolves.
- Recognize that your needs may change over time, requiring adjustments to your routine.

4. Establishing a Routine Schedule

a. Consistency is Key:

- Reaffirm the importance of consistency in your routine. Consistency fosters habit formation and maximizes the benefits of your practice.
- Consider aligning your routine with specific times of the day that resonate with your energy levels.

b. Flexibility and Adaptability:

- Embrace the idea of a flexible routine that can adapt to changes in your daily schedule.

- Acknowledge that life is dynamic, and your routine should be flexible enough to accommodate unexpected commitments.

5. Tracking Progress and Adjusting

a. Keeping a Journal:

- Dive deeper into the concept of a chair yoga journal, exploring ways to make it an integral part of your routine.
- Include reflections on how each session makes you feel physically, mentally, and emotionally.

b. Listening to Your Body:
- Develop a heightened awareness of your body's signals during and after each session.
- Be attuned to areas of tension, improvement, and areas that may require additional attention.

c. Periodic Evaluations:

- Incorporate periodic evaluations into your routine, reassessing your goals, progress, and the effectiveness of your routine.

- Consider seeking feedback from a yoga instructor or healthcare professional to ensure your routine aligns with your evolving needs.

Creating a structured chair yoga routine is a significant milestone in your wellness journey. By defining your goals, selecting poses, adapting them to your needs, establishing a routine schedule, and tracking your progress, you're not only establishing a habit but also fostering a deeper connection with your body and mind. In the upcoming chapter, we'll explore additional resources, including online classes, communities, and further reading, to enhance and deepen your chair yoga experience.

Chapter 6: Enhancing Your Chair Yoga Experience with Resources

Welcome to the gateway of resources designed to elevate your chair yoga experience. This chapter is a treasure trove of guidance, offering a plethora of options ranging from guided online classes to community engagement and further reading. Dive deep into these resources to enrich your chair yoga practice and embark on a journey of continuous growth.

1. Guided Online Classes

a.Selecting Reputable Platforms:

- **Explore a Variety of Platforms:** Begin your exploration with popular platforms like YouTube, where renowned yoga instructors often share free chair yoga sessions. Websites such as Yoga with Adriene or specialized yoga platforms also offer a diverse range of classes.

- **Instructor Specialization:** Look for instructors with expertise in chair yoga and experience working with diverse populations. Reading reviews and testimonials can provide insights into the effectiveness of their classes.

b. Diverse Class Lengths and Styles:

- **Customize Your Experience:** Consider your schedule and preferences when selecting classes. Opt for shorter sessions during busy days and longer, more immersive classes when time allows.

- **Experiment with Styles:** Chair yoga comes in various styles, from gentle flow to targeted sessions focusing on specific areas. Experiment with different styles to discover what resonates most with your body and goals.

c. Interactive Live Classes:

- **Real-Time Interaction:** Participate in live online classes for real-time interaction with the instructor. This dynamic experience fosters a sense of community and allows for personalized guidance.

- **Local Offerings:** Check local yoga studios or community centers for live chair yoga classes. This not only supports local businesses but also provides an opportunity to connect with like-minded individuals in your area.

2. Community Support and Engagement

a. Online Yoga Communities:

- **Virtual Connection:** Joining online communities dedicated to yoga creates a virtual space for sharing experiences, asking questions, and receiving support.

- **Platform Diversity:** Explore platforms like Reddit, Facebook groups, or specialized yoga forums. These spaces can serve as a source of inspiration and motivation as you connect with fellow chair yoga enthusiasts.

b. Local Yoga Classes and Workshops:

- **Local Connections:** Engage with your local community by exploring chair yoga classes or workshops. Community centers, senior centers, and yoga studios often offer specialized sessions.

- **In-Person Interaction:** Participating in local classes provides the unique opportunity to connect face-to-face with individuals who share a common interest in chair yoga.

c. Social Media Platforms:

- **Instagram and Beyond:** Leverage social media platforms like Instagram, where practitioners and instructors share insights, tips, and personal journeys related to chair yoga.

- Hashtags and Discoverability: Use relevant hashtags to discover and connect with a broader community. Social media can be a valuable tool for ongoing inspiration and community engagement.

3. Further Reading and Educational Resources

a. Books on Chair Yoga:

- In-Depth Exploration: Dive into dedicated books on chair yoga written by experts such as Lakshmi Voelker and Kristine Lee. These resources provide comprehensive instructions, pose variations, and the underlying philosophy of chair yoga.

- Incorporate Philosophy: Understanding the philosophy behind chair yoga can deepen your practice and offer a holistic perspective on its transformative potential.

b. Yoga Anatomy Guides:

- Holistic Understanding: Enhance your knowledge of yoga anatomy with resources like "The Key Muscles of Yoga" by Ray Long or "The Heart of Yoga" by T.K.V. Desikachar.

- Linking Anatomy to Practice: Connecting anatomy to your practice can provide valuable insights into how different poses impact your body and contribute to overall well-being.

c. Online Articles and Blogs:

- Regular Inspiration: Explore online articles and blogs dedicated to chair yoga. Many experienced practitioners and instructors share insights, practical tips, and personal experiences.

- Stay Updated: Subscribe to newsletters or bookmark reliable websites to stay updated on the latest developments, trends, and insights within the chair yoga community.

4. Creating a Home Practice Sanctuary

a. Choosing the Right Space:

- Personal Sanctuary: Designate a space at home specifically for your chair yoga practice. Ensure it is free from distractions and has ample natural light and ventilation.

- Create a Ritual: Establish a pre-practice ritual to signal the beginning of your chair yoga session. This could include lighting a candle or playing soft music to create a calming atmosphere.

b. Personalizing Your Space:

- **Inspirational Elements:** Add personal touches to your practice space, such as calming colors, motivational quotes, or a small altar with meaningful objects.

- **Positive Associations:** Personalizing your space creates a positive environment that encourages regular practice and contributes to a sense of well-being.

c. Investing in Props:

- **Enhanced Comfort:** Consider investing in yoga props like blocks, straps, or bolsters to enhance your practice.

- **Versatility of Props:** Props can be used to modify poses, provide additional support, and make your practice more comfortable and enjoyable. They add versatility to your chair yoga routine.

By delving into guided online classes, engaging with supportive communities, exploring further reading and educational resources, and creating a dedicated practice space, you are enriching your chair yoga journey. As we move toward the final chapter, let's summarize the key takeaways and offer words of encouragement. The transformative power of chair yoga awaits, and your commitment to this practice is a testament to your dedication to well-being.

Chapter 7: Embracing the Transformative Journey

Welcome to the culminating chapter of "Chair Yoga for Elders Over 60." Your commitment to this transformative journey is a testament to your dedication to well-being. As we reflect on the key takeaways from our exploration, let's delve deeper into the nuances of chair yoga and offer an abundance of encouragement for the ongoing path ahead.

1. Reflecting on Your Chair Yoga Journey

a. Celebrating Progress:

- Take a comprehensive look at your journey, celebrating not only physical advancements but also the mental and emotional shifts that chair yoga has catalyzed in your life.

- Consider creating a personal progress journal, noting specific milestones, moments of joy, and any challenges you've overcome.

b. Self-Discovery Through Practice:

- Delve into the profound self-discovery that occurs through chair yoga. Reflect on how your awareness of breath, body, and emotions has deepened over time.
- Consider journaling about any newfound insights into your own habits, reactions, or thought patterns that chair yoga has illuminated.

c. Adaptability and Growth:

- Explore the adaptability and growth you've experienced. Chair yoga is not just about physical flexibility; it's about cultivating a flexible mindset and nurturing personal growth.
- Embrace challenges as opportunities for learning and recognize that growth often happens in the spaces where you step out of your comfort zone.

2. Incorporating Chair Yoga Into Daily Life

a. Consistency is Key:

- Reinforce the notion that consistency is the cornerstone of a fruitful chair yoga practice. Consistent, regular practice, even if brief, yields cumulative benefits over time.

- Encourage the integration of chair yoga into your daily routine, making it a non-negotiable aspect of your self-care regimen.

b. Integrating Mindfulness:

- Deepen the integration of mindfulness beyond the mat. Encourage the application of mindfulness principles in daily activities, fostering a sense of presence in every moment.

- Share practical tips for incorporating mindful breathing or body awareness during routine tasks, enhancing overall awareness.

c. Sharing the Practice:

- Discuss the joy of sharing chair yoga with others. Consider organizing chair yoga sessions with friends, family, or community members.
- Emphasize the communal aspects of chair yoga, highlighting the potential for creating a supportive network of individuals sharing in the practice.

3. Continuing Your Chair Yoga Exploration

a. Exploring Advanced Poses:

- If practitioners feel ready, encourage the exploration of more advanced chair yoga poses. Provide guidance on how to gradually incorporate these poses, ensuring safety and enjoyment.

- Discuss the mental and physical benefits of challenging oneself, fostering a sense of accomplishment and resilience.

b. Expanding Your Practice:

- Advocate for the expansion of one's practice beyond chair yoga. Suggest complementary practices such as seated meditation, gentle stretching routines, or even exploring other styles of yoga.

- Emphasize the interconnectedness of various wellness practices, contributing to a holistic approach to health.

c. Staying Informed:

- Stress the importance of staying informed about the evolving field of chair yoga. Encourage practitioners to follow reputable instructors, join online communities, and attend workshops or events.

- Share recommendations for reputable websites, podcasts, or social media accounts that regularly provide updates on chair yoga trends and developments.

4. Fostering a Positive Mindset

a. Gratitude for Your Body:

- Deepen the practice of gratitude for one's body. Guide practitioners in developing a daily gratitude ritual, expressing appreciation for the body's resilience and capabilities.
- Explore the psychological benefits of gratitude, including increased positivity and resilience in the face of challenges.

b. Embracing Challenges:

- Discuss the transformative potential embedded in challenges. Encourage practitioners to embrace difficulties as opportunities for growth, emphasizing the resilience that arises from navigating obstacles.

- Share personal stories or anecdotes that highlight the positive outcomes that can emerge from facing challenges head-on.

c. Loving-Kindness Toward Yourself:

- Dive into the concept of self-compassion. Introduce loving-kindness meditation or affirmations as tools for fostering a compassionate attitude toward oneself.

- Emphasize the importance of self-care and self-acceptance in the chair yoga journey.

5. Acknowledging the Transformative Power

a. Mind-Body Connection:

- Deepen the understanding of the mind-body connection nurtured by chair yoga. Illustrate how the integration of breath, movement, and mindfulness contributes to a profound sense of well-being.

- Discuss the physiological benefits of the mind-body connection, including improved stress management, immune function, and overall mental health.

b. Well-Being Beyond the Mat:

- Explore the ripple effects of chair yoga beyond the mat. Discuss how the positive impact on mental health, emotional well-being, and overall quality of life transcends the confines of a yoga session.

- Share stories or testimonials from individuals who have experienced transformative changes in their lives through chair yoga.

c. Continuing the Journey:

- Conclude with an invitation to view chair yoga as a lifelong journey. Emphasize that each breath, movement, and moment of mindfulness contributes to a cumulative and enduring sense of well-being.

- Express optimism about the limitless possibilities for growth and self-discovery that lie ahead on the chair yoga journey.

As we conclude our exploration of chair yoga for elders over 60, let gratitude fill your heart for the commitment you've shown to your well-being. May your chair yoga practice continue to be a source of joy, vitality, and transformation. The journey is ongoing, and each step is a testament to your dedication to a healthier and more mindful life.

Thank you for embarking on this journey with "Chair Yoga for Elders Over 60." May your path be illuminated with wellness, mindfulness, and the enduring transformative power of chair yoga.

Chapter 8: Sustaining the Radiance: Ongoing Practices and Beyond

Welcome to the final chapter of "Chair Yoga for Elders Over 60." This chapter is designed to provide you with sustaining practices, tips for continuous growth, and insights into how chair yoga can become an enduring and enriching part of your life. As you read on, let the wisdom within these pages guide you on your journey towards sustained well-being.

1.Daily Chair Yoga Rituals

a. **Morning Awakening Sequence:**
   - Begin your day with a gentle chair yoga awakening sequence. Incorporate movements that stretch and invigorate your body, setting a positive tone for the day ahead.

- Emphasize the importance of connecting with your breath, fostering mindfulness from the moment you wake up.

b. Midday Refresh and Reset:

- Introduce a midday chair yoga routine to refresh and reset your energy. Focus on poses that combat sedentary stiffness, promoting circulation and mental clarity.
- Encourage short mindful breaks throughout the day, utilizing chair yoga techniques to maintain a sense of balance and well-being.

c. Evening Relaxation Ritual:

- Wind down in the evening with a chair yoga sequence designed for relaxation. Incorporate gentle stretches, calming breathwork, and mindfulness practices to prepare your body for restful sleep.
- Establish a consistent evening routine to signal the transition from the busyness of the day to a peaceful state of mind.

2. Expanding Your Chair Yoga Repertoire

a. Exploration of New Poses:

- Continue expanding your repertoire of chair yoga poses. Regularly introduce new poses to keep your practice engaging and to target different muscle groups.
- Explore online resources, books, or attend local workshops to discover fresh perspectives and pose variations.

b. Incorporating Props Creatively:

- Experiment with creative ways to use props in your chair yoga practice. Props can enhance your experience by providing support, stability, and facilitating deeper stretches.

- Share tips on how to adapt everyday household items into makeshift props to make your practice accessible and versatile.

c. Mindfulness Walks and Outdoor Practices:

- Extend your chair yoga practice beyond the confines of your home. Enjoy mindful walks in nature, incorporating seated or standing chair yoga poses in serene outdoor settings.
- Embrace the therapeutic benefits of connecting with nature and infuse your practice with the beauty and tranquility of the outdoors.

3. Holistic Well-Being Practices

a. Nutrition and Chair Yoga:
- Explore the intersection of chair yoga and nutrition. Discuss mindful eating practices, emphasizing the importance of nourishing your body with wholesome, balanced meals.

- Provide insights into how conscious eating aligns with the principles of chair yoga, promoting overall well-being.

b. Mindful Breathing Throughout the Day

- Integrate mindful breathing into various aspects of your daily life. Whether at work, during chores, or in moments of stress, use your breath as an anchor to cultivate a calm and centered mindset.
- Share simple breath-awareness exercises that can be seamlessly incorporated into any situation.

c. Gratitude Journaling:

- Foster a sense of gratitude through journaling. Establish a daily gratitude practice, noting down moments of joy, achievements, or things you are thankful for.
- Reflect on how cultivating gratitude aligns with the holistic philosophy of chair yoga,

promoting a positive outlook and emotional well-being.

4. Connecting with the Chair Yoga Community

a. Online Communities and Challenges:

- Stay connected with the chair yoga community through online platforms. Join challenges, participate in virtual events, and engage with like-minded individuals.

- Share your own ney and insights, inspiring others while drawing inspiration from the diverse experiences within the chair yoga community.

b. Local Workshops and Events:

- Attend local chair yoga workshops or events. Engage with your community, meet fellow practitioners, and deepen your understanding of chair yoga in a collaborative setting.

- Share information about upcoming local events or establish a group within your community to organize regular chair yoga gatherings.

c. Mentoring and Sharing Wisdom:

- Consider mentoring others who are new to chair yoga. Share your experiences, offer guidance, and create a supportive space for mutual growth.

- Cultivate a sense of community where practitioners of all levels can exchange wisdom, fostering a spirit of shared learning and encouragement.

5. Long-Term Well-Being and Lifelong Learning

a. Chair Yoga Teacher Training

- Explore the possibility of chair yoga teacher training if you have a deep passion for the practice. Becoming a certified chair yoga instructor allows you to share the benefits with a broader audience.

- Highlight the various avenues available for teacher training, both online and in-person, and the potential for personal growth through the teaching journey.

b.Continued Education and Workshops:

- Commit to lifelong learning in the field of chair yoga. Attend advanced workshops, enroll in courses, and seek out educational opportunities that align with your evolving interests.

- Emphasize the richness that ongoing education brings to your practice, allowing you to continuously deepen your understanding of chair yoga.

c. Community Outreach and Service:

- Explore ways to give back to your community through chair yoga. Consider offering free sessions to local seniors, organizing chair yoga events in community spaces, or collaborating with healthcare facilities.

- Share stories of how chair yoga can be a powerful tool for community outreach and service, contributing to the well-being of diverse populations.

As you embrace the sustaining practices outlined in this chapter, remember that chair yoga is not just a series of poses; it's a holistic philosophy that can enrich every aspect of your life. Continue to explore, learn, and share the transformative power of chair yoga, knowing that your journey is an ongoing, evolving, and infinitely rewarding process.

Chapter 9: Resources for Further Exploration

Congratulations on completing "Chair Yoga for Elders Over 60." As you embark on the ongoing journey of chair yoga, this chapter provides a curated list of resources to deepen your understanding, explore new perspectives, and connect with the broader chair yoga community. Whether you're seeking additional reading, online classes, or communities for support, this chapter is your guide to further exploration.

1. Recommended Reading

a. Essential Chair Yoga Books

- **Chair Yoga:** Sit, Stretch, and Strengthen Your Way to a Happier, Healthier You* by Kristin McGee.

- **Lakshmi Voelker Chair Yoga: The Sitting Mountain Series*** by Lakshmi Voelker.

- **The Key Muscles of Yoga** by Ray Long - Explores yoga anatomy and its application to various poses, including chair yoga.

b. Mindfulness and Wellness:

The Miracle of Mindfulness by Thich Nhat Hanh - A classic guide to mindfulness practices.

The Whole-Body Breathing by Sue Hitzmann - Focuses on breathwork and its impact on overall well-being.

c. Yoga Philosophy and Lifestyle:

- *The Heart of Yoga* by T.K.V. Desikachar - A comprehensive exploration of yoga philosophy and practice.

The Four Agreements by Don Miguel Ruiz - Offers practical wisdom for personal freedom and a fulfilling life.

2. Online Classes and Platforms

a. Guided Chair Yoga Sessions:

- Explore platforms such as YouTube and DoYogaWithMe for a variety of chair yoga sessions led by experienced instructors.

b. Live Classes and Communities:

- Check out platforms like Yoga International for live classes, workshops, and a supportive community.
- Consider local yoga studios that offer in-person or virtual chair yoga classes.

c. Teacher Training and Certification:

- Look into organizations like Yoga Alliance and YogaEd for information on chair yoga teacher training programs and certifications.

3. Online Communities and Forums

a. Social Media Groups:
- Join chair yoga communities on social media platforms like Facebook and Instagram to connect with practitioners and instructors.

b. Forums and Discussion Boards
- Engage in discussions related to chair yoga on forums like Yoga Forums and Reddit's Yoga Community.

4. Additional Learning and Workshops

a. Continuing Education Programs:

- Explore online workshops and articles offered by Yoga Journal for continuous learning in yoga.

- Consider checking resources provided by The International Association of Yoga Therapists (IAYT) for additional workshops.

b. Local Events and Gatherings:

- Attend local yoga studios, community centers, and wellness events for chair yoga workshops and gatherings.

- Explore health and wellness expos or conferences for opportunities to deepen your understanding of chair yoga.

5. Community Outreach and Volunteering

a. Senior Centers and Community Organizations

- Connect with local senior centers or community organizations to volunteer your chair yoga skills.
- Offer free chair yoga sessions to underserved communities, contributing to the well-being of diverse populations.

b. Collaborate with Healthcare Professionals:

- Reach out to healthcare professionals and inquire about opportunities to integrate chair yoga into wellness programs.
- Explore partnerships with physical therapists, occupational therapists, and healthcare providers to support individuals on their healing journey.

As you continue your chair yoga journey, may these resources serve as beacons of inspiration, knowledge, and connection. Remember that the path of wellness is a lifelong exploration, and with each resource, you have the opportunity to deepen your practice and share the transformative benefits of chair yoga with others.

Thank you for joining the journey of "Chair Yoga for Elders Over 60." May your ongoing exploration be filled with joy, growth, and the radiant well-being that chair yoga offers.

<u>CONCLUSION</u>

Congratulations on reaching the end of "Chair Yoga for Elders Over 60." This journey has been a shared exploration of well-being, mindfulness, and the transformative power of chair yoga. As you reflect on the wisdom imparted throughout this book, remember that this conclusion is not an end but a new beginning—a beginning filled with possibilities for continued growth, self-discovery, and radiant well-being.

Chair yoga is more than a series of poses; it's a philosophy that invites you to embrace each moment with mindfulness, kindness, and a deep connection to your body and breath. Whether you are just starting your chair yoga practice or have been on this journey for some time, know that the path is ever-evolving, offering you the opportunity to rediscover the joy of movement, the peace of breath, and the resilience of your spirit.

As you integrate chair yoga into your daily life, consider the following:

1. **Consistency is Key:** Small, regular sessions of chair yoga can have a profound impact over time. Approach your practice with a sense of commitment, and let each breath become a reminder of your dedication to your well-being.

2. **Mindful Living:** Extend the principles of mindfulness cultivated during chair yoga to all aspects of your life. Be present in each moment, savoring the simple joys, and approaching challenges with a centered mind.

3. **Share the Joy:** Consider sharing chair yoga with friends, family, or your community. The benefits of chair yoga are universal, and introducing others to this practice can create a positive ripple effect, fostering well-being in your social circle.

4. **Explore and Learn:** Keep the spirit of exploration alive. Continue to explore new poses, expand your practice, and delve into the rich philosophy of chair yoga. Lifelong learning is a gateway to continued growth and self-discovery.

5. **Connect with the Community:** Whether through online platforms, local events, or community outreach, stay connected with the chair yoga community. Share your journey, learn

from others, and contribute to the collective well-being.

Remember, your chair yoga journey is a personal odyssey, and every breath, every movement, and every mindful moment contributes to your well-being. The practice is not confined to the mat; it is a way of living that embraces the potential for transformation in every aspect of your life.

Thank you for being a part of "Chair Yoga for Elders Over 60." May your journey be filled with ongoing discovery, radiant health, and the enduring joy that comes from the practice of chair yoga.

Namaste.

Reader Reviews

We invite you to share your thoughts and experiences with "Chair Yoga for Elders Over 60." Your reviews are invaluable in helping others discover the transformative benefits of chair yoga and guiding them on their wellness journey. Whether you are a beginner or an experienced practitioner, we appreciate your insights and reflections.

How to Submit Your Review:

1. **Title:** Craft a title that reflects your overall impression or a specific aspect of the book that stood out to you.
2. **Rating:** Assign a rating out of 5 stars to express your overall satisfaction with the book.
3. **Review Text:** Share your thoughts, experiences, and any specific benefits you've gained from practicing chair yoga based on the book's guidance.

4. Recommendation: Would you recommend this book to others? Why or why not?

5. Your Name or Pseudonym: Sign your review with your real name or a pseudonym, whichever you're comfortable with.

Feel free to include details about how the book has influenced your well-being, any favorite chapters or exercises, and whether it met your expectations. Your reviews contribute to a collective understanding of the book's impact and help build a supportive community around chair yoga.

Thank you for taking the time to share your review. Your words have the power to inspire and guide others on their chair yoga journey.

Namaste.

www.ingramcontent.com/pod-product-compliance
Lightning Source LLC
Chambersburg PA
CBHW070837260726
48660CB00005B/2068